Understanding and Managing Tourette Syndrome

A comprehensive guide to help individuals with Tourette syndrome gain control over tics

Introduction

In a world where diversity is celebrated, it is vital that we extend our understanding and empathy to those who navigate life with conditions that set them apart from the norm. Tourette Syndrome (TS) is one such condition, a neurological disorder characterized by involuntary motor and vocal tics that often begin in childhood. Despite its prevalence, TS remains shrouded in myths and misconceptions, leading to stigma and isolation for those who live with it.

This book, "Understanding and Managing Tourette Syndrome: A Comprehensive Guide," seeks to shed light on the complexities of TS, offering knowledge, compassion, and practical guidance to individuals, families, educators, and healthcare professionals. By delving deep into the world of TS, we aim to foster a more inclusive and informed society where individuals with TS can thrive.

TS presents unique challenges, but it is also marked by resilience, creativity, and strength. Through these pages, you will embark on a journey of discovery. We will explore the origins of TS, its diagnosis, and the everyday experiences of those who live with it. We will discuss treatment options, strategies for managing tics, and the importance of building a support network. We will also address the coexisting conditions often associated with TS and provide insights into advocacy and community support.

Table of contents

Chapter 1

What is Tourette Syndrome?

In the realm of neurological conditions, Tourette Syndrome (TS) stands as a distinctive and often misunderstood phenomenon. To embark on our journey of understanding and managing TS, we must first delve into the fundamental question: What is Tourette Syndrome?

Defining Tourette Syndrome

At its core, Tourette Syndrome is a neurological disorder characterized by repetitive, involuntary movements and sounds known as tics. These tics can manifest as motor tics (sudden, rapid, and repetitive muscle movements) or vocal tics (uncontrolled vocalizations or sounds). While tics can vary widely in their frequency and severity, they are the hallmark of TS.

A Brief Historical Perspective

The history of TS dates back to the 19th century when the French neurologist Dr. Georges Gilles de la Tourette first described the condition in 1885. Dr. Tourette's pioneering work shed light on the disorder, and it eventually came to bear his name. Since then, significant progress has been made in understanding TS, though many mysteries still remain.

The Prevalence of TS

Tourette Syndrome is more common than one might think. It is estimated that approximately 1 in 100 children between the ages of 5 and 17 in the United States have been diagnosed with TS or a related tic disorder. Moreover, TS knows no geographical boundaries, affecting individuals of diverse backgrounds worldwide. It is crucial to recognize that TS does not discriminate based on age, gender, or ethnicity.

Distinguishing TS from Other Tic Disorders

While TS is the most well-known tic disorder, it is not the only one. Distinguishing between TS and other tic disorders is essential for accurate diagnosis and treatment. Some individuals may experience transient tics, which are temporary and typically resolve on their own. Chronic tic disorders involve tics lasting for over a year, but they may not meet all the criteria for TS.

Key Takeaways

In this introductory chapter, we have laid the foundation for our exploration of Tourette Syndrome. We have defined TS as a neurological disorder characterized by tics, explored its historical context, and highlighted its prevalence. Furthermore, we've touched upon the importance of distinguishing TS from other tic disorders.

Chapter 2

The Causes and Diagnosis of TS

In our exploration of Tourette Syndrome (TS), we now turn our attention to the intriguing questions of what causes this condition and how it is diagnosed. Understanding the origins of TS and the process of diagnosis is crucial in providing the best support and care for individuals affected by it.

Unraveling the Complex Causes of TS

The exact cause of TS remains an area of ongoing research and study. However, it is widely believed to be a complex interplay of genetic, neurological, and environmental factors. Here are some key aspects to consider:

Genetic Predisposition:
- Evidence suggests that genetics play a significant role in TS. Studies have shown that TS tends to run in families, and individuals with a family history of the disorder are at a higher risk of developing it.

Neurological Factors:
- Abnormalities in certain brain regions and
neurotransmitter systems have been linked to TS. In
particular, the basal ganglia and frontal cortex are
believed to play a crucial role in the manifestation of tics.

Environmental Factors:
- While genetics and neurobiology lay the foundation,
environmental factors may trigger or exacerbate TS
symptoms. Factors such as prenatal exposure to toxins,
infections, or trauma have been explored in research.

The Diagnostic Process

Diagnosing Tourette Syndrome is a multifaceted process
that requires careful evaluation by healthcare
professionals. It is essential to recognize the signs and
symptoms of TS and distinguish them from other
conditions that may present with similar features. Here
are the key components of the diagnostic process:

Diagnostic Criteria:
- TS is diagnosed based on specific criteria outlined in
medical guidelines. These criteria typically include the
presence of both motor and vocal tics that have
persisted for at least one year, with symptom onset
before the age of 18.

Clinical Assessment:
- Healthcare professionals, such as neurologists,
psychiatrists, or pediatricians, conduct a thorough

clinical assessment. They gather a detailed medical history, perform physical examinations, and may use diagnostic tools to rule out other conditions.

Observation and Documentation:
- Observing the frequency, duration, and complexity of tics is essential for diagnosis. Careful documentation of tic patterns and their impact on daily life aids in the diagnostic process.

Addressing Common Misconceptions

As we delve into the causes and diagnosis of TS, it is essential to dispel common misconceptions. TS is not solely a result of stress, anxiety, or emotional disturbance, as some may believe. It is a neurological condition with a biological basis.

Key Takeaways

In this chapter, we have delved into the complex factors that contribute to Tourette Syndrome. We've explored the role of genetics, neurology, and environmental factors in the development of TS. Additionally, we've outlined the diagnostic process, emphasizing the importance of accurate assessment by healthcare professionals.

Chapter 3

Living with TS: Challenges and Stigma

Tourette Syndrome (TS) is more than just a collection of tics; it is a condition that can profoundly affect the lives of those who experience it. In this chapter, we will delve into the challenges individuals with TS often face, including the pervasive stigma that can accompany this condition.

The Daily Struggles

Living with TS can be a daily challenge, as individuals contend with the unpredictability of tics. Here are some of the key difficulties faced by those with TS:

Social and Interpersonal Challenges:
- Social situations can be particularly daunting. Individuals with TS may worry about how their tics will be perceived by others, leading to anxiety and social withdrawal.
- Bullying and teasing can be common, especially during childhood and adolescence when peers may not understand TS.

Academic and Occupational Challenges:
- TS can impact concentration and focus, making it challenging for students to excel academically. It may also affect career choices and job performance.
- The fear of tics occurring during important tasks, such as exams or presentations, can add additional stress.

Emotional and Psychological Impact:
- Living with a condition that draws attention to oneself can lead to feelings of embarrassment and low self-esteem.
- Coping with the challenges of TS can contribute to anxiety and depression for some individuals.

Dispelling Misconceptions

Unfortunately, TS is often surrounded by misconceptions that further compound the challenges faced by those with the condition. It is crucial to address and correct these misconceptions to create a more understanding and supportive society:

TS is Not a Choice:
- Many mistakenly believe that individuals with TS can simply control their tics if they try hard enough. In reality, tics are involuntary and difficult to suppress.

TS is Not a Sign of Intellectual Disability:
- TS has no bearing on a person's intelligence. Many individuals with TS are highly intelligent and capable of achieving academic and professional success.

TS is Not a Behavioral Problem:
- TS is a neurological condition, not a behavioral issue. Punishment or discipline is not an effective way to manage tics.

The Power of Understanding and Support

While living with TS presents challenges, it is essential to recognize the remarkable strength and resilience of individuals who navigate this journey. The power of understanding and support from family, friends, educators, and healthcare professionals cannot be underestimated.

Key Takeaways

In this chapter, we have explored the myriad challenges that individuals with Tourette Syndrome face in their daily lives. From social and academic hurdles to emotional and psychological impact, TS can be a complex and demanding condition to manage.

As we continue our journey through this book, we will delve into strategies for providing effective support and empowering individuals with TS to thrive. By fostering a compassionate and informed environment, we can begin to break down the barriers and stigma that individuals with TS encounter, allowing them to lead fulfilling lives true to their unique selves.

Chapter 4

Treatment Options

In our quest to understand and manage Tourette Syndrome (TS), one of the crucial aspects to explore is the array of treatment options available to individuals with TS. While there is no one-size-fits-all solution, this chapter will provide insights into various approaches and strategies for managing TS symptoms and improving overall quality of life.

A Multidimensional Approach

Managing TS often requires a multidimensional approach that may include medical, behavioral, and supportive interventions. The choice of treatment depends on the severity of symptoms and individual needs.

Behavioral Therapy:
Comprehensive Behavioral Intervention for Tics (CBIT):
CBIT is a structured, evidence-based behavioral therapy designed to help individuals with TS manage their tics. It involves techniques such as tic awareness, competing responses, and habit reversal training. CBIT is typically administered by trained therapists.

Medications:
Antipsychotic Medications:
In some cases, healthcare providers may prescribe antipsychotic medications to reduce the frequency and severity of tics. Common medications include haloperidol, risperidone, and aripiprazole. However, these medications may have side effects that need to be carefully monitored.

Supportive Therapies:
-**Psychotherapy**: Therapy, such as cognitive-behavioral therapy (CBT), can help individuals manage stress, anxiety, and any emotional challenges associated with TS.
-**Occupational and Speech Therapy**:
These therapies can be beneficial for addressing functional difficulties related to TS, such as motor coordination or speech difficulties.

Weighing the Pros and Cons

Deciding on the appropriate treatment for TS requires careful consideration of the potential benefits and drawbacks. Here are some key factors to weigh:

Benefits of Treatment:
- **Reduction in Tic Severity**:
Effective treatment can lead to a decrease in the frequency and intensity of tics, improving overall quality of life.

- Enhanced Daily Functioning:
By managing tics and associated challenges, individuals with TS can better focus on their studies, work, and social interactions.

Drawbacks and Considerations:

- Side Effects:
Some medications may have side effects, which need to be monitored and managed in consultation with healthcare professionals.

- Individual Variability:
TS is a highly variable condition, and what works for one person may not work for another. Treatment plans need to be tailored to individual needs.

The Importance of Informed Decision-Making

It is crucial for individuals and their families to engage in informed decision-making when it comes to TS treatment. This involves open communication with healthcare providers, understanding the risks and benefits of various interventions, and considering the individual's goals and preferences.

Key Takeaways

In this chapter, we've explored the various treatment options available for Tourette Syndrome. From behavioral therapy and medications to supportive interventions, there are approaches to address the unique needs of individuals with TS.

Chapter 5

Strategies for Managing Tics

Living with Tourette Syndrome (TS) often involves navigating the challenges presented by tics—those involuntary motor and vocal behaviors that define the condition. In this chapter, we will explore practical strategies and techniques to help individuals with TS manage their tics and lead more fulfilling lives.

Tic Awareness and Self-Monitoring

Understanding one's tics is the first step in managing them effectively. Tic awareness involves recognizing the triggers, frequency, and patterns of tics. Self-monitoring can be a powerful tool for gaining insight into one's condition. Some strategies include:

- **Keeping a Tic Diary**:
 Recording when and where tics occur, as well as any preceding sensations or feelings, can help identify patterns and triggers.
- **Recognizing the "Premonitory Urge"**:
Many individuals with TS experience an uncomfortable sensation or urge before a tic. Learning to recognize

and manage this premonitory urge is essential for tic control.

Habit Reversal Training (HRT)

Habit Reversal Training is a structured behavioral therapy designed to help individuals with TS manage their tics. It focuses on replacing tics with more socially acceptable, less disruptive movements or sounds. Key components of HRT include:

- **Awareness Training**: Identifying tics and their triggers.
- **Competing Response**: Developing an alternative, voluntary action that is incompatible with the tic.
- **Relaxation Techniques:** Learning relaxation methods to reduce the urge to tic.

Environmental Modifications

Creating a supportive environment can make a significant difference in managing tics. Consider these strategies:

- **Minimize Stress:** High stress levels can exacerbate tics. Encourage relaxation techniques and stress-reduction activities.
- **Classroom or Workplace Accommodations**: For students and employees, working with educators or employers to make accommodations can help reduce tic-related stress.

Medication Management

In some cases, individuals with TS may opt for medication to help control tics. Medications are typically considered when tics significantly impact daily functioning. However, it's essential to be aware of potential side effects and work closely with healthcare providers to find the right medication and dosage.

Support Systems

Having a strong support system is invaluable for individuals with TS. Friends, family members, and support groups can provide emotional support and understanding. Here are some ways to build and maintain support systems:

- **Educate Loved Ones:** Help friends and family understand TS and its challenges so that they can provide better support.
- **Join Support Groups**: Engage with local or online TS support groups to connect with others who share similar experiences.

Patience and Self-Compassion

Above all, it's crucial for individuals with TS to practice patience and self-compassion. Managing tics can be challenging, and there will be ups and downs along the way. Remember that TS does not define a person's worth or potential, and everyone's journey is unique.

Key Takeaways

In this chapter, we've explored practical strategies for managing tics associated with Tourette Syndrome. From increasing tic awareness and implementing habit reversal training to creating supportive environments and seeking support from loved ones, there are numerous ways to enhance one's ability to manage tics effectively.

Chapter 6

Supporting Children and Adolescents with TS

Tourette Syndrome (TS) often manifests in childhood, and its impact on children and adolescents can be profound. In this chapter, we will explore the unique challenges faced by young individuals with TS and provide guidance for parents, teachers, and caregivers on creating a supportive environment.

Understanding TS in Children

Recognizing TS in children can be challenging, as tics are often mistaken for normal childhood behaviors or dismissed as passing phases. It is crucial to be aware of the following:

- **Early Onset**: TS typically begins between the ages of 5 and 10, and early diagnosis is essential for timely intervention and support.
- **Variable Course**: Tics may change in frequency and severity over time. Understanding the fluctuating nature of tics is essential.

The Role of Parents and Caregivers

Parents and caregivers play a pivotal role in supporting children with TS. Here are key strategies for providing effective support:

- **Education**: Learn about TS to better understand your child's condition and its challenges.
- **Open Communication**: Encourage your child to express their feelings and concerns, fostering an environment of trust.
- **Advocacy**: Advocate for your child's needs in educational and healthcare settings, ensuring they receive appropriate accommodations and support.

Navigating the Educational Environment

The school environment can pose unique challenges for children with TS. Effective collaboration between parents, teachers, and school staff is essential:

- **Individualized Education Plan (IEP):** Work with the school to create an IEP tailored to your child's needs, which may include accommodations for tics and associated difficulties.
- **Teacher Awareness**: Educate teachers about TS, its symptoms, and the importance of patience and understanding.

- **Peer Education:** Consider classroom discussions or presentations about TS to promote empathy and reduce stigma among peers.

Empowering Adolescents with TS

As children with TS transition into adolescence, they face additional challenges related to self-identity, independence, and social acceptance. Here's how to empower adolescents with TS:

- **Self-Advocacy**: Encourage your child to become their own advocate, teaching them to communicate their needs and educate others about TS.
- **Building Resilience**: Help your child develop coping strategies to manage stress and anxiety, which can exacerbate tics.
- **Exploring Interests**: Support your child's interests and hobbies, helping them build self-confidence and a sense of identity beyond TS.

Addressing Coexisting Conditions

It's common for children and adolescents with TS to have coexisting conditions such as Attention-Deficit/Hyperactivity Disorder (ADHD) or Obsessive-Compulsive Disorder (OCD). Identifying and addressing these conditions is essential for comprehensive care.

Key Takeaways

In this chapter, we've explored the unique challenges faced by children and adolescents with Tourette Syndrome. By understanding the early onset of TS, the role of parents and caregivers, the educational environment, and the importance of empowering adolescents, we can create a more supportive and inclusive environment for young individuals affected by TS.

Chapter 7

TS and Coexisting Conditions

Tourette Syndrome (TS) rarely exists in isolation. Many individuals with TS also contend with coexisting conditions that can complicate their experiences and care. In this chapter, we will explore common coexisting conditions, the challenges they pose, and how a multidisciplinary approach can provide comprehensive care.

Recognizing Coexisting Conditions

It is not uncommon for individuals with TS to have one or more coexisting conditions, including but not limited to:

Attention-Deficit/Hyperactivity Disorder (ADHD):
- ADHD is characterized by symptoms of inattention, hyperactivity, and impulsivity. It often coexists with TS, making it important to address both conditions simultaneously.

Obsessive-Compulsive Disorder (OCD):
- OCD involves intrusive, repetitive thoughts (obsessions) and ritualistic behaviors (compulsions). It can be challenging when OCD symptoms intertwine with TS tics.

Anxiety Disorders:
- Anxiety disorders, such as generalized anxiety disorder or social anxiety disorder, are common among individuals with TS due to the stress and social challenges associated with the condition.

Learning Disabilities:
- Some individuals with TS may have learning disabilities that affect their academic performance and require additional educational support.

The Complex Interplay

Coexisting conditions can interact with TS in complex ways, amplifying challenges and affecting overall well-being. For example:

- OCD rituals may be mistaken for tics, leading to misunderstandings.
- Anxiety can exacerbate both tics and coexisting conditions.
- ADHD symptoms may interfere with concentration and academic performance.

A Multidisciplinary Approach

To address the complexities of TS and coexisting conditions, a multidisciplinary approach is often necessary:

- **Medical Management:** Healthcare providers may prescribe medications to manage coexisting conditions, such as ADHD or OCD. Careful monitoring is essential to balance symptom relief and potential side effects.

- **Behavioral Therapy:** Evidence-based therapies, such as cognitive-behavioral therapy (CBT), can be effective in treating coexisting conditions like OCD or anxiety.

- **Educational Support:** Collaborate with educators and specialists to develop tailored educational plans, including accommodations and modifications for students with TS and learning disabilities.

- **Family Support:** Engage in family therapy or support groups to address the impact of TS and coexisting conditions on family dynamics.

Tailoring Treatment Plans

Each individual with TS and coexisting conditions is unique, and treatment plans should be tailored to their specific needs and challenges. It may require trial and error to find the most effective interventions.

Key Takeaways

In this chapter, we've explored the complex landscape of coexisting conditions that often accompany Tourette Syndrome. Understanding the interactions between TS and these conditions is crucial for providing comprehensive care.

Chapter 8

Advocacy and Community Support

Advocacy and community support are vital components of understanding and managing Tourette Syndrome (TS). In this chapter, we will explore the importance of advocacy, the role of support groups, and the power of coming together to create a more inclusive and informed society for individuals with TS.

The Power of Advocacy

Advocacy involves raising awareness, promoting understanding, and fighting for the rights and well-being of individuals with TS. Here's why advocacy is essential:

Reducing Stigma:
- Advocacy efforts aim to dispel myths and misconceptions about TS, combatting the stigma often associated with the condition.

Access to Resources:
- Advocacy can lead to improved access to healthcare, education, and support services for individuals with TS.

Promoting Research:
- Advocacy organizations often fund research to better understand TS and develop more effective treatments.

Advocacy at Different Levels

Advocacy can occur at various levels, from individual and family advocacy to broader community and legislative efforts:

- **Individual Advocacy:** Advocating for your own needs or those of your child, such as requesting accommodations in school or the workplace.
- **Family Advocacy**: Joining forces with other families affected by TS to collectively advocate for improved services and support.
- **Community Advocacy**: Participating in local awareness campaigns and events to educate the public about TS.
- **Legislative Advocacy**: Lobbying for legislation that benefits individuals with TS, such as anti-discrimination laws or funding for research.

The Role of Support Groups

Support groups are invaluable for individuals with TS and their families. They provide a sense of belonging, understanding, and shared experience. Key aspects of support groups include:

- **Emotional Support**: Sharing experiences, challenges, and successes with others who understand TS can be immensely comforting.

- **Information Sharing:** Support groups offer a platform to exchange information about treatments, resources, and strategies for managing TS.
- **Advocacy and Awareness**: Many support groups engage in advocacy efforts to raise awareness and improve the lives of individuals with TS.

Navigating Online Communities

The digital age has expanded the reach of support and advocacy efforts. Online communities, forums, and social media groups can connect individuals with TS to a global network of support and information.

Encouraging Self-Advocacy

Advocacy doesn't have to be limited to external efforts. Empowering individuals with TS to become self-advocates is equally important. Encouraging them to understand their condition, communicate their needs, and advocate for themselves fosters independence and resilience.

Key Takeaways

In this chapter, we've explored the essential role of advocacy and community support in understanding and managing Tourette Syndrome. Advocacy efforts can help reduce stigma, improve access to resources, and promote research, while support groups offer emotional support, information sharing, and a sense of belonging.

Chapter 9

Living a Fulfilling Life with TS

Tourette Syndrome (TS) is not a barrier to leading a fulfilling and successful life. In this final chapter, we will focus on the potential for individuals with TS to thrive, highlighting examples of achievement, resilience, and empowerment. We will encourage readers to embrace their uniqueness and pursue their passions, no matter how unique they may be.

The Journey of Self-Discovery

Embracing life with TS often begins with self-discovery. It's essential for individuals with TS to:

- **Accept Themselves**: Recognize that TS is just one aspect of who they are and that it does not define their worth or potential.
- **Set Personal Goals:** Encourage individuals to set goals based on their interests and passions, whether they are academic, creative, or personal.

Role Models and Inspiration

Throughout history, many individuals with TS have achieved remarkable success in various fields. Sharing these stories can inspire others:

- **Artists and Musicians**: Many renowned artists and musicians, such as Mozart and Samuel Johnson, are believed to have had TS.
- **Athletes**: Some athletes, like soccer player Tim Howard and basketball player Mahmoud Abdul-Rauf, have overcome TS to excel in their sports.
- **Advocates**: Individuals like Tim Shriver, Chairman of Special Olympics, have become powerful advocates for individuals with TS and other neurological conditions.

Building Resilience

Resilience is a key trait that can help individuals with TS face life's challenges:

- **Coping Strategies**: Encourage the development of healthy coping strategies, such as mindfulness, meditation, or physical activity, to manage stress and anxiety.
- **Positive Self-Talk:** Teach individuals to challenge negative self-perceptions and replace them with positive affirmations.

The Importance of a Support Network

Family, friends, educators, and support groups can play a pivotal role in helping individuals with TS thrive:

- **Encourage Communication**: Open and honest communication with loved ones fosters understanding and empathy.
- **Celebrate Achievements**: Acknowledge and celebrate every accomplishment, no matter how small, to boost self-esteem and motivation.

Embracing Uniqueness

Every individual with TS has a unique combination of strengths, talents, and interests. Encourage readers to:

- **Pursue Passions:** Explore and embrace hobbies and interests that bring joy and fulfillment.
- **Educate Others**: Share knowledge about TS with others to foster understanding and acceptance.

Final Thoughts

In closing, this book has been a journey through the world of Tourette Syndrome—its challenges, complexities, and the potential for growth and fulfillment. TS may present unique hurdles, but it is by no means a barrier to living a life rich in meaning, achievement, and happiness.

As you move forward, remember that understanding and managing TS is not just about symptom control; it is about embracing one's individuality, fostering resilience, and pursuing dreams with unwavering determination. By doing so, individuals with TS can contribute to a more inclusive, compassionate, and informed world—one that recognizes the inherent value and potential in every person, regardless of their neurodiversity.

The journey may have its ups and downs, but with the right support, self-acceptance, and determination, individuals with TS can indeed lead fulfilling and purposeful lives.

Conclusion

Our exploration of Tourette Syndrome (TS) has taken us on a profound journey—from understanding its origins to recognizing the unique challenges individuals with TS face, from discovering treatment options to advocating for change, and finally, to embracing the potential for a fulfilling life.

Throughout this book, we've strived to shed light on TS, dispel myths, and foster empathy and support for those affected by this neurological condition. We've emphasized the importance of knowledge, compassion, and resilience in the face of adversity.

As we conclude this journey, we leave you with a few essential takeaways:

- TS is a neurological condition characterized by tics—repetitive, involuntary movements and sounds. It often begins in childhood but continues into adulthood for many individuals.

- Early diagnosis and intervention are crucial to providing individuals with TS the support they need to thrive. Understanding the causes, symptoms, and diagnosis of TS is a critical first step.

- Living with TS can be challenging, with individuals facing a range of difficulties, including social stigma, academic and occupational hurdles, and emotional struggles. However, with understanding and support, these challenges can be overcome.

- Treatment options for TS include behavioral therapy, medication, and supportive interventions. The choice of treatment depends on individual needs and should be tailored to the specific challenges posed by TS.

- Coexisting conditions, such as ADHD, OCD, and anxiety, are common among individuals with TS. Recognizing and addressing these conditions is essential for comprehensive care.

- Advocacy and community support are powerful tools in breaking down the barriers and stigma that individuals with TS often encounter. By advocating for awareness, understanding, and improved services, we can create a more inclusive and compassionate society.

- TS does not define an individual's worth or potential. Embracing uniqueness, setting personal goals, and building resilience can empower individuals with TS to lead fulfilling lives.

As you embark on your journey beyond these pages, remember that knowledge is the key to understanding and empathy. By sharing what you've learned about TS, advocating for change, and offering support to those affected by the condition, you contribute to a world that values diversity and celebrates the strength and resilience of every individual.

Thank you for joining us on this exploration of Tourette Syndrome. May your newfound understanding and compassion inspire positive change and brighter futures for all individuals with TS and their families.